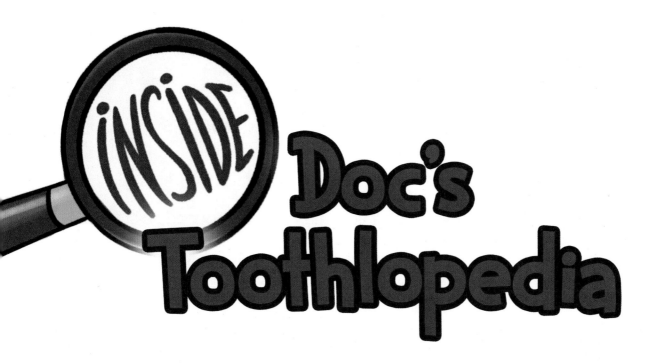

The Dental Visit

By Dr. Patricia M.A. Simons

Volume 2, F-N

Inside Doc's Toothlopedia
The Dental Visit

Volume 2, F–N

Copyright © 2023 by Patricia M.A. Simons, DDS, MS

Published by: Toothlopedia, LLC, USA
www.toothlopedia.com

Designs — Original Concept, Story, and Characters: Patricia Simons, DDS, MS

Illustrator: Alyssa Erin
www.alyssaerin.com

Made in the USA
ISBN 979-8-9884503-1-3
First Edition, 2023

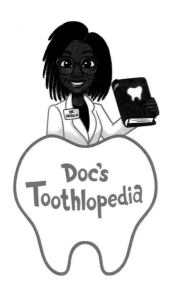

Doc's Toothlopedia

Hello, everyone! My name is Dr. Patricia, and I am a general dentist. I aim to provide the best care to patients of all ages and educate the community. I am passionate about learning and want to spread my knowledge to all of you so that you can share what you learn with family and friends! Growing up, I loved reading encyclopedias (uhn-sai-kluh-PEE-dee-uhs) and still do! Book volumes are full of exciting facts and fun things to learn!

Doc's Toothlopedia (tooth-low-PEE-dee-uh) is a dental book you can learn from, just like an encyclopedia! Each volume will build off what you learned in the previous book. Now that you are reading this, you are officially part of Team Toothlopedia! Congrats!

I encourage parents or loved ones to read this book together with children until the words become more familiar. I recommend reading Volume I of Doc's Toothlopedia prior to this book and to children ages six and up. You can also enjoy coloring in Doc's Toothlopedia Coloring and Activities books!

Toothlopedia and beyond!
Dr. Patricia

This book is dedicated to the Adesanya and Simons families for all their support over the years.

"Welcome back, everyone!" said Dr. Patricia as each member of Team Toothlopedia walked into the dental office and high-fived each other. She waved goodbye to the family members who dropped them off.

"It is great to see all of you again! In order to make sure everyone is here, I made special Team Toothlopedia name tags for each of you."

"Cool!" shouted the children as they placed the name tags on their shirts.

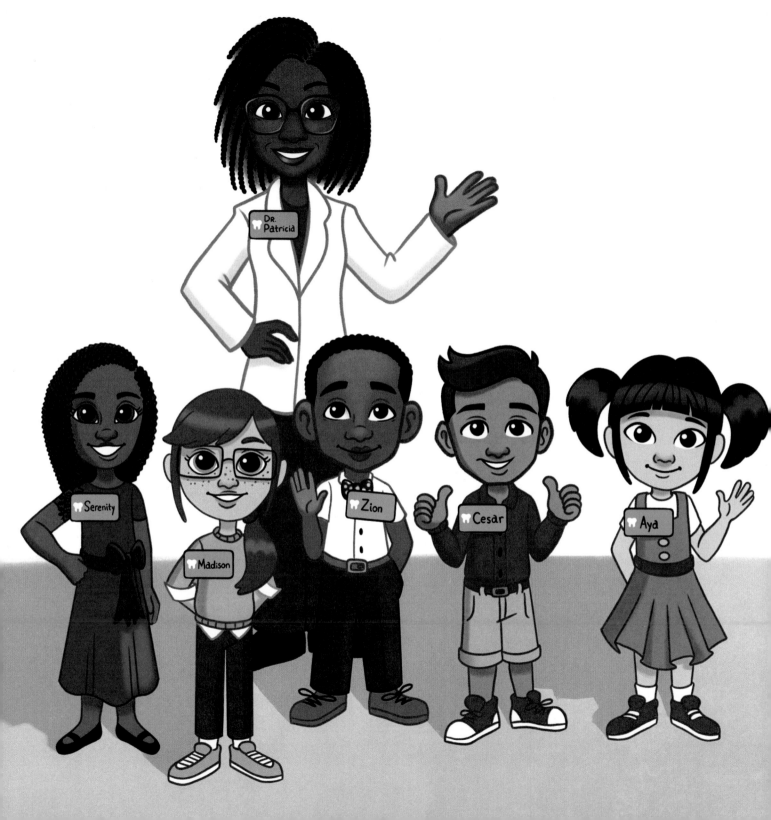

Aya skipped to a stack of dental books on the table
and picked up the Toothlopedia.

"Is it time to start learning the dental words of the day?"
asked Aya as she held the book out to the group.

"Let's do it!" said everyone.

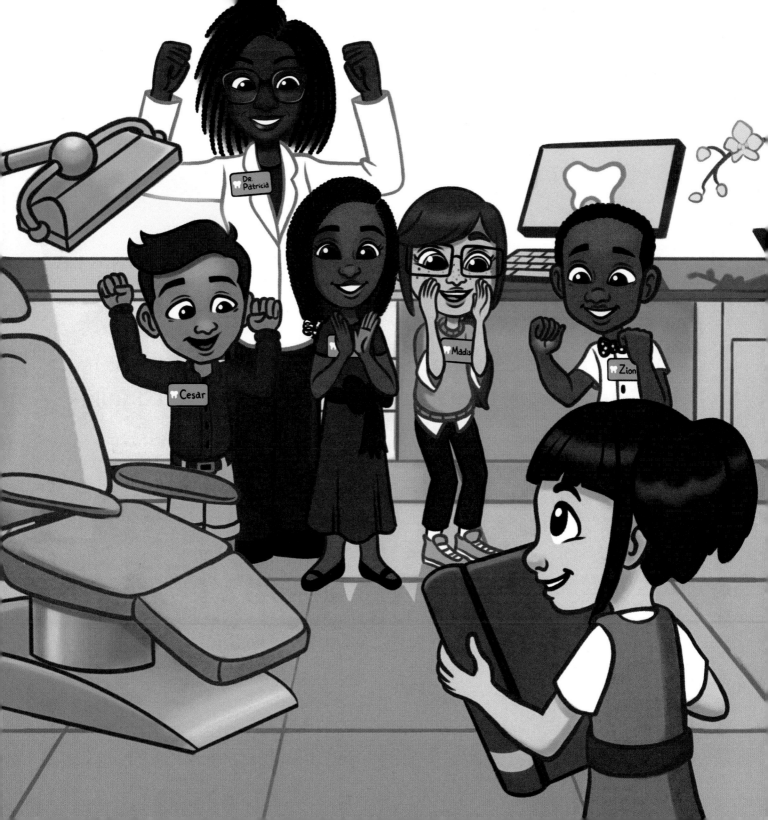

Dr. Patricia pulled out her special magnifying glass from her pocket to help see all the words for the day.

As Dr. Patricia raised the magnifying glass, it came to life. "Well, hello, everyone! It is good to see all of you again!" said Mr. Magni.

"Hi, Mr. Magni!" shouted everyone.

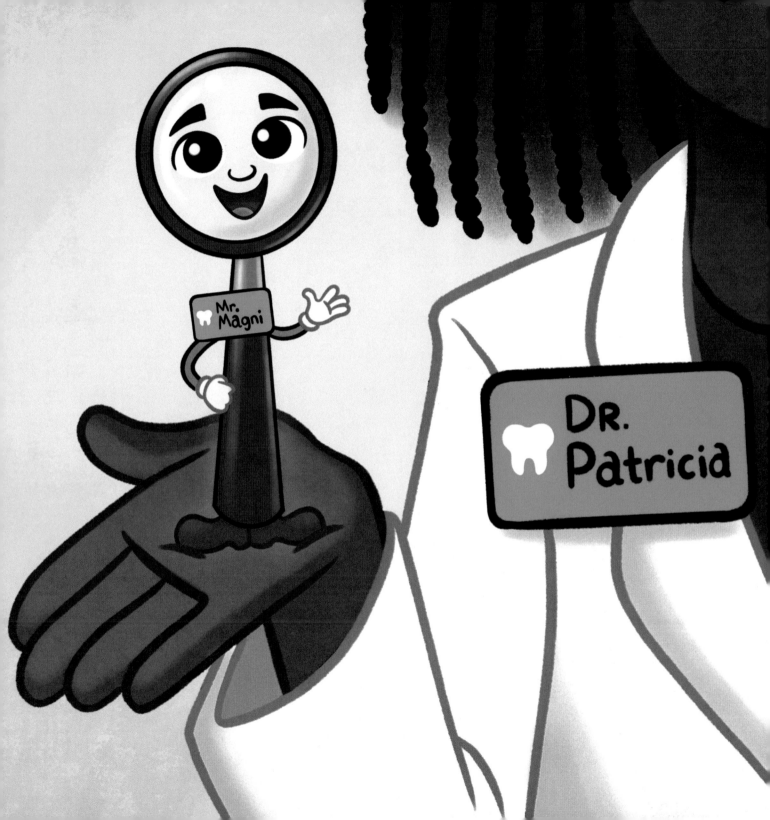

Team Toothlopedia gathered around,
and as Aya opened the book, it glowed.

When the children looked through Mr. Magni,
the words became large, and magical pictures appeared.

Aya flipped the pages to the first word of the day.

"Filling," said Aya.

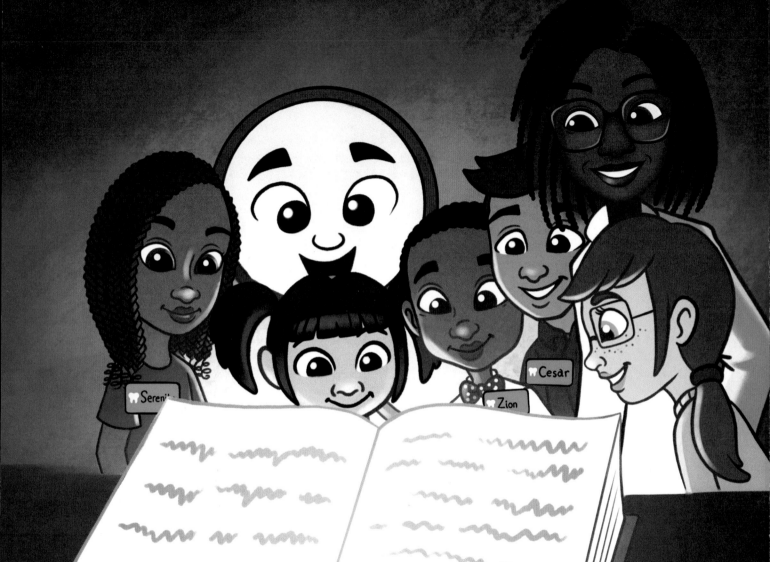

Filling
(FI-luhng)

Reminder from Volume 1: Sticky and slimy stuff called plaque (plak) is full of germs (bad bacteria like S.mutans), can break down a tooth, and form a hole called a cavity.

Please do not worry if you have a cavity!
A dentist, like Dr. Patricia, will come to the rescue and treat your tooth with a **filling**.
The dentist might use "sleepy juice" to put your tooth to sleep so that you are comfy.
The dentist will clean the icky stuff out of the cavity and fill the hole with a special material that will protect your tooth and keep it strong!

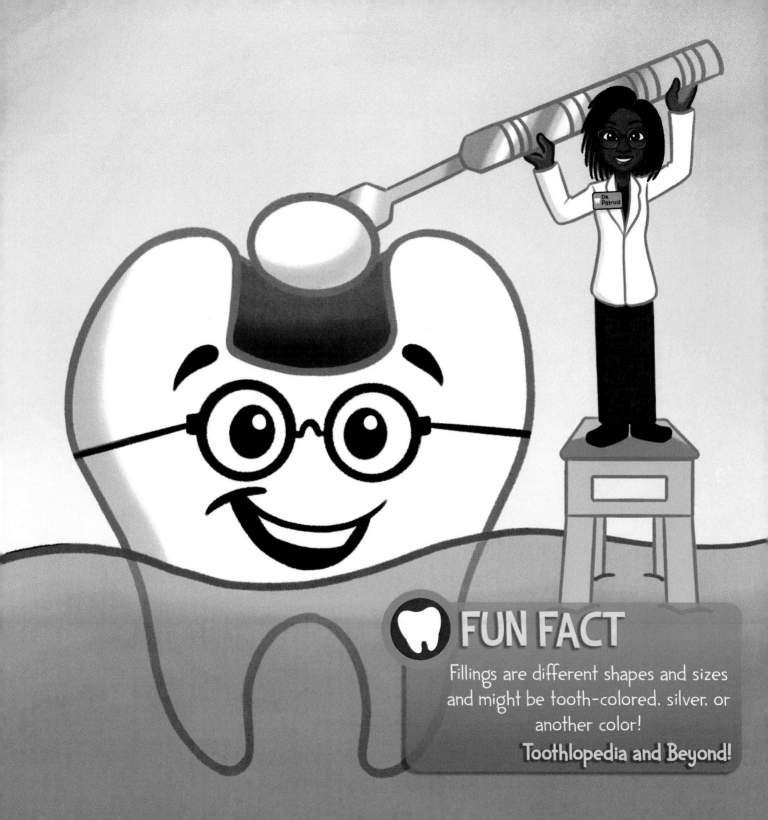

FUN FACT

Fillings are different shapes and sizes and might be tooth-colored, silver, or another color!

Toothlopedia and Beyond!

Floss
(flaas)

Do you ever feel like you have food stuck between your teeth? That might be because sticky and slimy plaque (plak) is hanging out there! Ewwwwww!

So, how do you clean between your teeth? The answer is **<u>floss</u>**.

<u>Floss</u> is a silky string that slides between your teeth to clean where your toothbrush can't reach.

Using **<u>floss</u>** once a day keeps both your teeth and gums healthy.

Keep reading along to learn about "gums!"

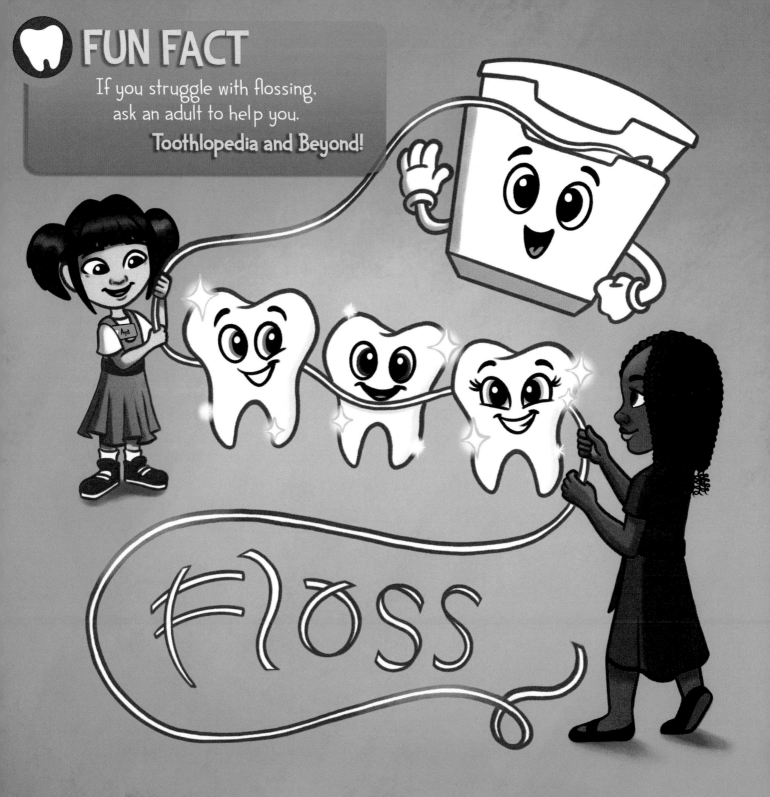

FUN FACT

If you struggle with flossing, ask an adult to help you.

Toothlopedia and Beyond!

Fluoride
(FLAW-ride)

When you visit the dental office,
a special paste made of **fluoride** may
be painted all over your teeth after they are
squeaky clean to prevent cavities.

Think of **fluoride** as "vitamins" to
help your teeth stay strong and healthy.

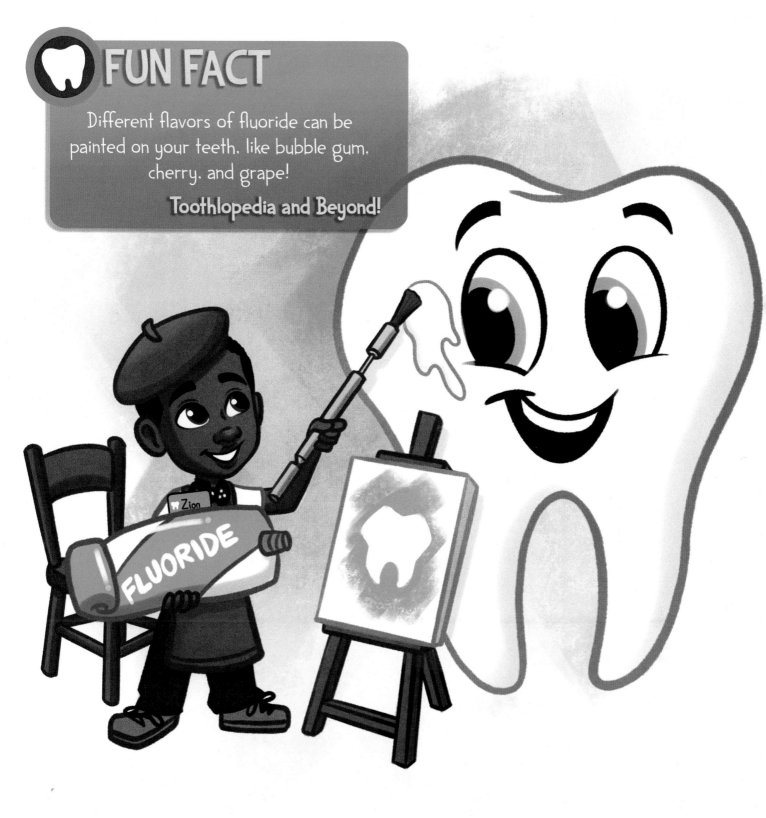

FUN FACT

Different flavors of fluoride can be painted on your teeth, like bubble gum, cherry, and grape!

Toothlopedia and Beyond!

Gums
(guhmz)

Don't get too excited!
This is not bubble gum!

Look into your mirror and smile very big.
The pink areas around your teeth are called **gums.**

Gums cover the bones in your mouth and the
bottom part of your teeth.
Gums also protect your teeth and
help to hold them in place.

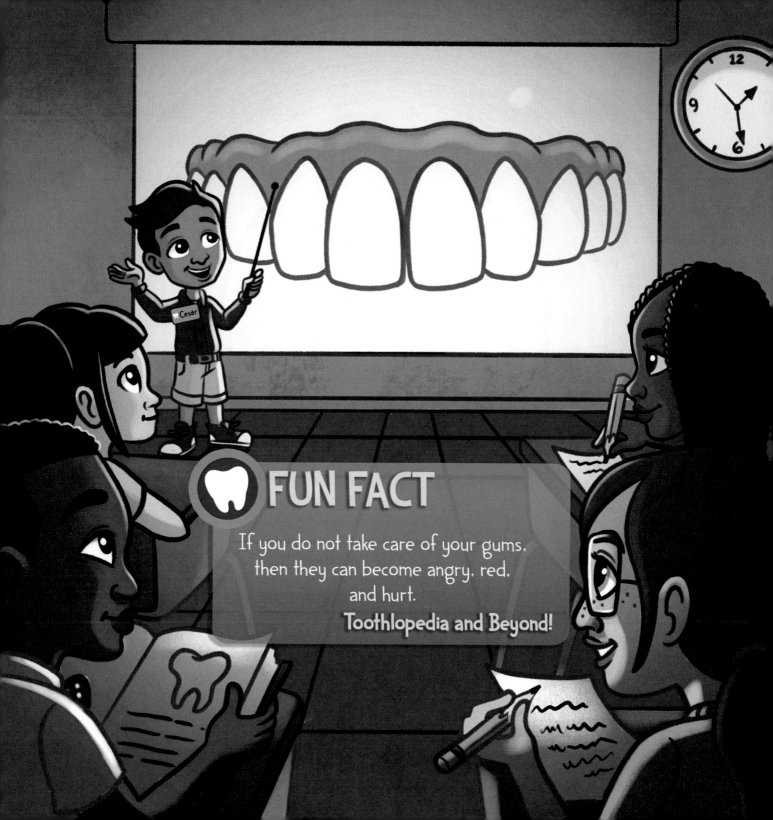

Hygienist
(hai-JEH-nuhst)

A **hygienist** works in the dental office with the dentist.

Hygienists have special training to clean your teeth and keep your gums healthy. When you go to a dental office, the **hygienist** softly removes any sticky plaque (plak) from areas you can't reach. They have neat tools to get the job done, and your teeth will be clean and shiny after!

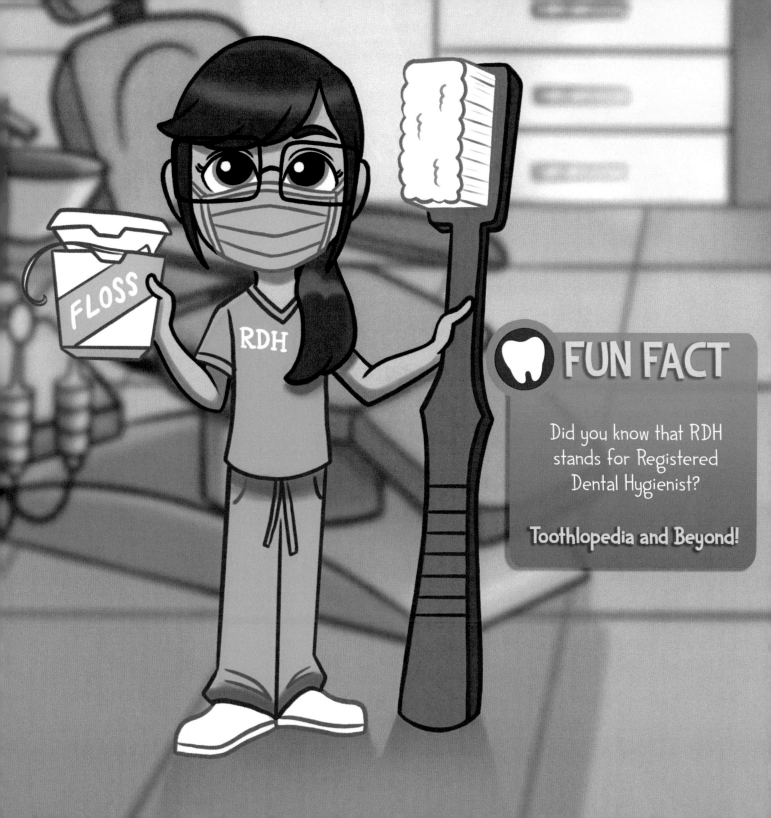

Incisors
(uhn-SAI-zrz)

Time to look into your mirror again!

Do you see your four front teeth on the top and bottom of your mouth?

Those four front teeth are called **incisors**, and they are like tiny chisels used to cut and tear food!

When you bite into a sandwich, your **incisors** are the first to dig in!

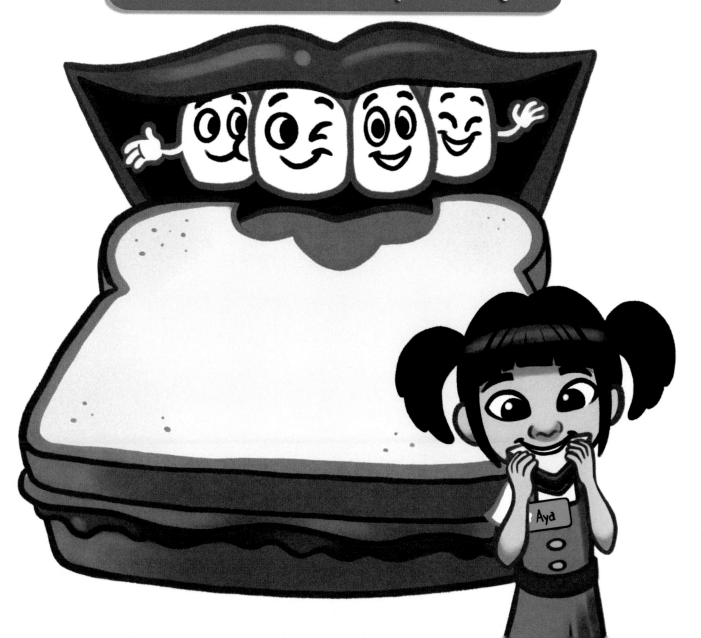

Jaws
(jaaz)

Think of your <u>jaws</u> as the bones your teeth are held in.

Since you have teeth on the top and bottom of your mouth, that means you have a top <u>jaw</u> and a bottom <u>jaw</u>.

When you move your bottom <u>jaw</u> up and down, you can open and close your mouth and chew your food!

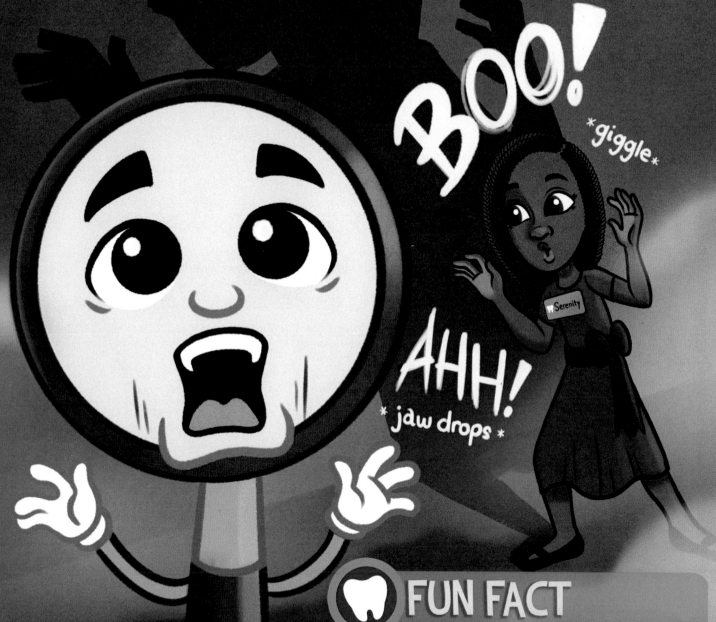

BOO!
giggle

AHH!
jaw drops

🦷 FUN FACT

If something startles or scares you, your jaw may "drop" like Mr. Magni's.

Toothlopedia and Beyond!

Kit

(kit)

The special tools that take care of your teeth are placed into a dental **kit** so that the tools can be cleaned, put in order, and stored away after an appointment.

Think of it as a toolbox that holds different items. Some tools in a dental **kit** check and count your teeth. There may be a tool to check your gums too!

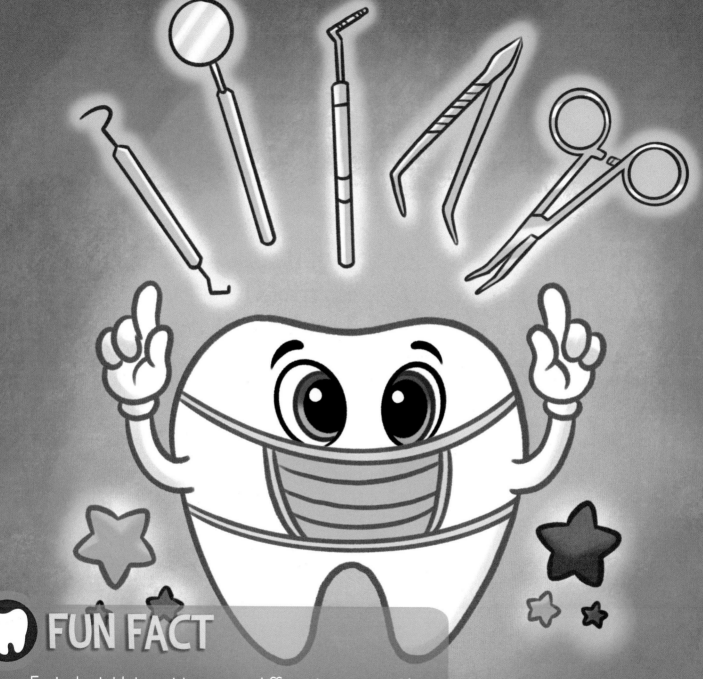

FUN FACT

Each dental kit might serve a different purpose, like cleaning your teeth, applying fillings, wiggling a loose tooth out, and more.

Toothlopedia and Beyond!

Letters
(LEH-trz)

Sing! A, B, C, D, E, F, G . . .

Those are the <u>letters</u> of the alphabet!

Each of your baby teeth has a <u>letter</u> that

belongs to it. If you hear your dentist call out a

<u>letter</u> of the alphabet, they are likely talking

about your baby tooth!

The name of each baby tooth on the top right of

your mouth starts with "A" and ends with "J" on

the left side.

Then your bottom teeth on the left side of

your mouth start with "K" and end

with "T" on the right side.

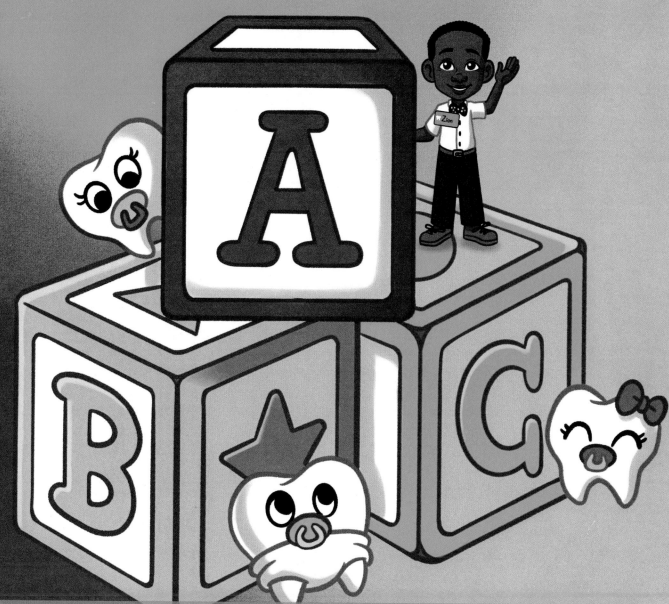

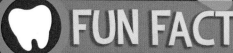 FUN FACT

Do you remember from Volume 1 that you can have up to twenty baby teeth in your mouth? That also means you can have twenty "letter" names for each tooth!

Toothlopedia and Beyond!

Lost Tooth
(laast tooth)

Losing a baby tooth might seem scary,
but it is a good thing!
Your baby teeth are holding spaces for your
"adult" teeth to come in as you grow up.
Your adult teeth can last forever if you
take good care of them!
So, if you lost a tooth, it is truly OK! See if another
tooth is already peeking through your gums!
Celebrate your **lost tooth** with your
family and friends! Cesar is celebrating his
lost tooth with you!

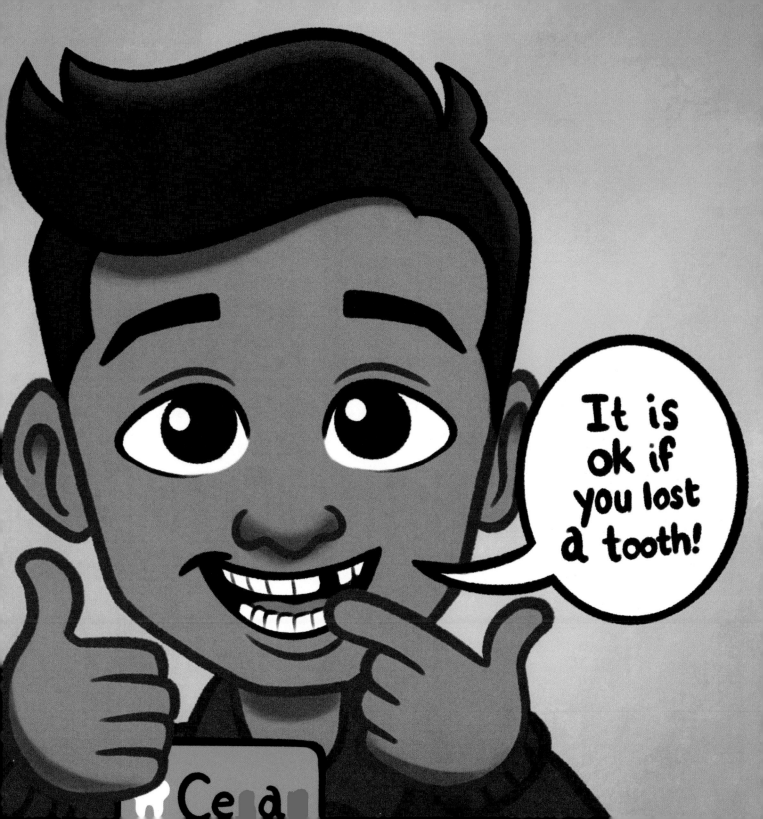

Molars
(MOW-lrz)

Can you feel the back teeth in your mouth with your tongue?

They should feel different from your front teeth! Those large back teeth on the top and bottom of your mouth are called **molars**.

Molars have round points and flat areas to help crush and grind your food after you bite into it.

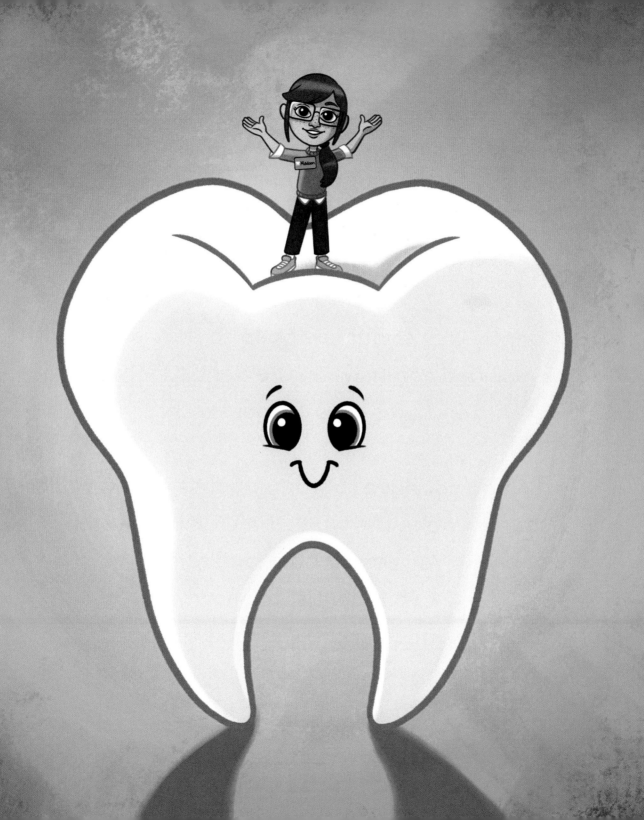

Mouth Prop
(mowth praap)

A **mouth prop** is a "chair" for your
teeth to sit in.
It gently keeps your jaw open so that your mouth
is nice and comfy when the dentist or hygienist
takes care of your teeth.

You do not have to worry about holding your
mouth open the whole time all by yourself!
You can sit back and relax!
Ask your dentist to show you a
mouth prop the next time
you go!

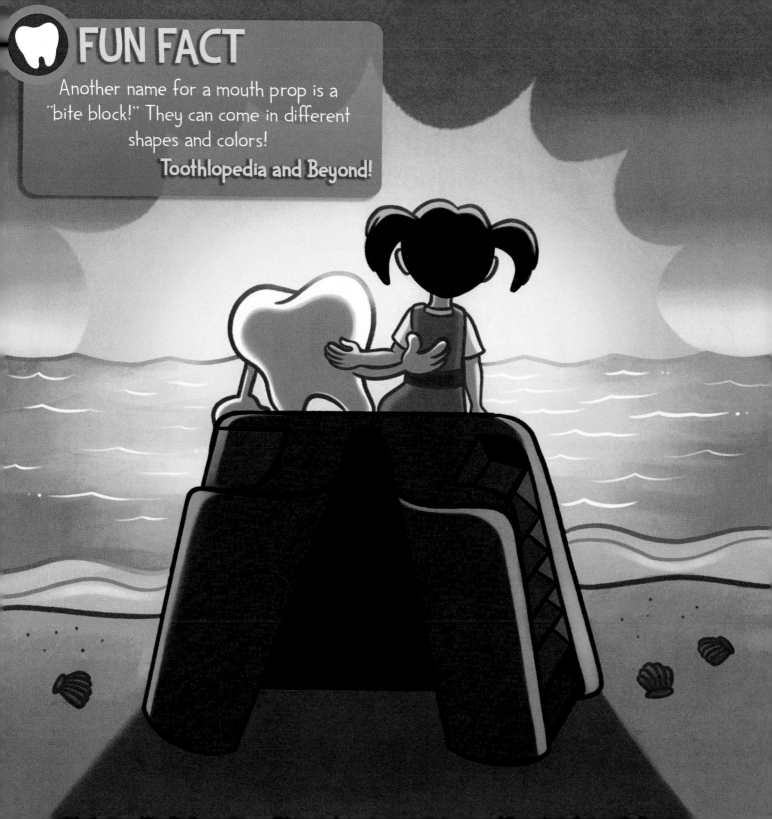

Numbers
(NUHM-brz)

Earlier, you learned about your baby teeth having letters as names. Guess what? Your adult teeth have names too, but this time they are **numbers**.

When all your baby teeth are gone and your adult teeth grow in, they can start with names of **number** 1 all the way to **number** 32!

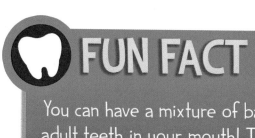

FUN FACT

You can have a mixture of baby teeth AND adult teeth in your mouth! That means you can have both letters and numbers at the same time to name your teeth!

Toothlopedia and Beyond!

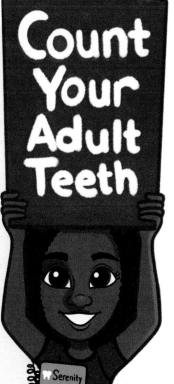

Count Your Adult Teeth

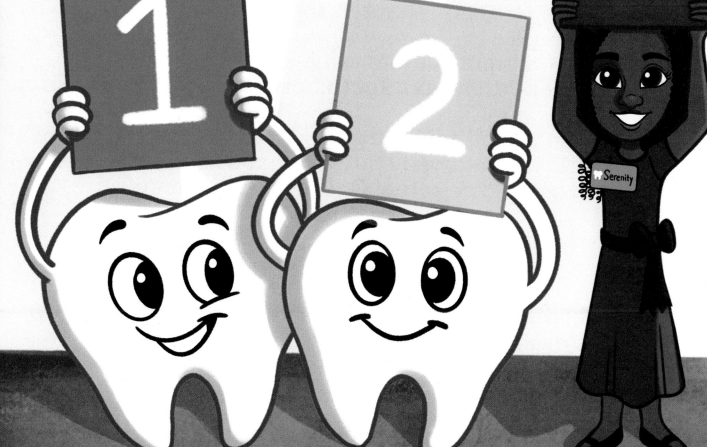

"That is all for today, Team Toothlopedia,"
said Dr. Patricia as she closed the book.

"Great job today with learning all the words!
Now, it is time to share what you learned
with your family and friends!"

"Woohoo!" shouted the children.

"Can we bring our family members next time
so they can be part of Team Toothlopedia too?" asked Cesar.

"Yes, of course you all can! They are all part of the team too!"
said Dr. Patricia. "Everybody put your hands in. Toothlopedia
and beyond on three! One . . . two . . . three!"

"Toothlopedia and beyond!" shouted everyone
as they threw their hands in the air.

The children rushed outside to meet their families,
excited to tell them about their day.

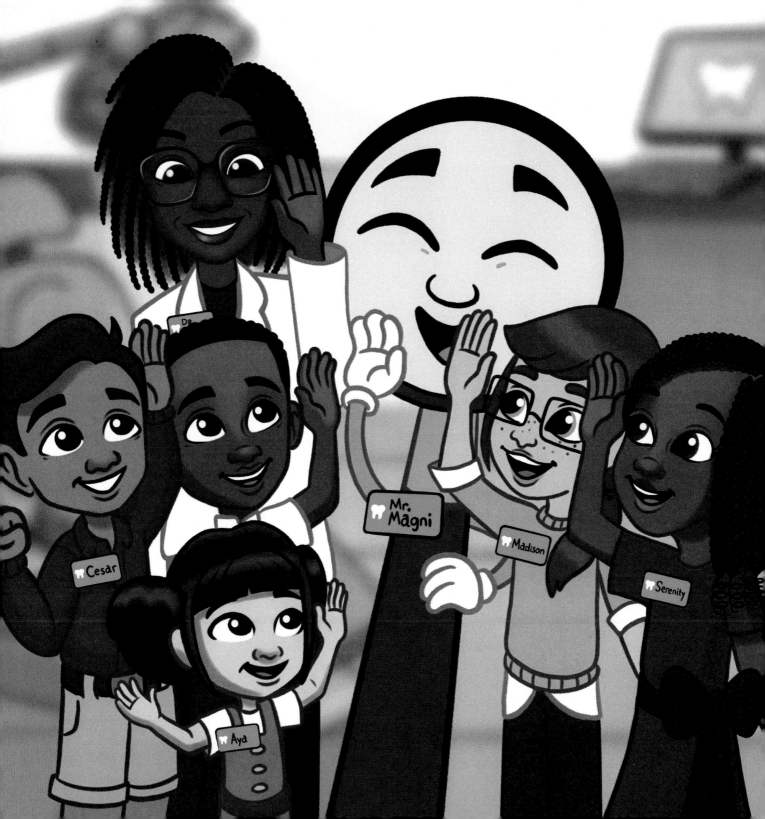

Toothlopedia Words Learned

Filling	Incisors	Molars
Floss	Jaws	Mouth Prop
Fluoride	Kit	Numbers
Gums	Letters	
Hygienist	Lost Tooth	

In Volume 3, we will start with learning <u>ortho</u> and <u>palate</u>!

Toothlopedia Family Quiz

Answers are at the bottom of the page.

Question 1: What kind of "names" do baby teeth have?

_____

Question 2: What kind of "names" do adult teeth have?

_____

Question 3: Which type of teeth are the biggest teeth in the mouth? _____

Question 4: How many times a day does Dr. Patricia want you to floss? _____

Question 5: Did you learn something today? _____
If so, give yourself a pat on the back!

20240989R00024